Competency Based Logbook in

Pharmacology

for Second Professional MBBS

4

As per the latest CBME Guidelines | Competency Based
Undergraduate Curriculum for the Indian Medical Graduate

Name: _____

Roll No.: _____ University Registration No.: _____

Date of Admission: _____

Permanent Address: _____

E-mail ID: _____ Batch: _____

Mobile No.: _____

Competency Based Logbook in

Pharmacology

for Second Professional MBBS

As per the latest CBME Guidelines | Competency Based
Undergraduate Curriculum for the Indian Medical Graduate

4

Niket Verma MBBS, MD

Assistant Professor
Department of General Medicine
Army College of Medical Sciences
Delhi Cantt, New Delhi

Poonam Agrawal MBBS, MD (Biochemistry)

Professor and Head
Department of Biochemistry
Dr Baba Saheb Ambedkar Medical College
and Hospital
New Delhi

Deepti Chopra MD

Assistant Professor
Department of Pharmacology
Government Institute of Medical
Sciences, Greater Noida, UP

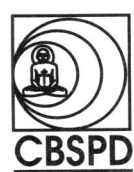

CBSPD

CBS Publishers & Distributors Pvt Ltd

New Delhi • Bengaluru • Chennai • Kochi • Kolkata • Lucknow • Mumbai
Hyderabad • Jharkhand • Nagpur • Patna • Pune • Uttarakhand

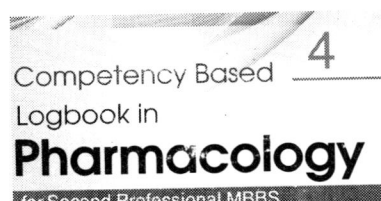

Competency Based 4

Logbook in

Pharmacology

for Second Professional MBBS

ISBN: 978-93-90709-48-9

Copyright © Authors and Publisher

First Edition: 2021
   Reprint: 2022, 2024 2025

Published by Satish Kumar Jain and produced by Varun Jain for

CBS Publishers & Distributors Pvt Ltd
4819/XI Prahlad Street, 24 Ansari Road, Daryaganj, New Delhi 110 002, India.
Ph: 011-23289259, 23266861   Website: www.cbspd.com
                                    e-mail: delhi@cbspd.com

Corporate Office: 204 FIE, Industrial Area, Patparganj, Delhi 110 092
Ph: 011-4934 4934   Fax: 011-4934 4935   e-mail: publishing@cbspd.com; publicity@cbspd.com

Branches

- **Bengaluru:** Seema House 2975, 17th Cross, K.R. Road, Banasankari 2nd Stage, Bengaluru 560 070, Karnataka, India
  Ph: +91-80-26771678/79   Fax: +91-80-26771680   e-mail: bangalore@cbspd.com
- **Chennai:** 7, Subbaraya Street, Shenoy Nagar, Chennai 600 030, Tamil Nadu, India
  Ph: +91-44-26680620, 26681266   Fax: +91-44-42032115   e-mail: chennai@cbspd.com
- **Kochi:** 42/1325, 1326, Power House Road, Opp KSEB, Power House, Ernakulam, Kochi, 682 018, Kerala, India
  Ph: +91-484-4059061-65/67   Fax: +91-484-4059065   e-mail: kochi@cbspd.com
- **Kolkata:** 147, Hind Ceramics Compound, 1st Floor, Nilgunj Road, Belghoria, Kolkata 700 056, West Bengal, India
  Ph: +91-33-2563355/56   e-mail: kolkata@cbspd.com
- **Lucknow:** Basement, Khushnuma Complex, 7-Meerabai Marg (Behind Jawahar Bhawan), Lucknow 226 001, UP, India
  Ph: +91-522-4000032   e-mail: tiwari.lucknow@cbspd.com
- **Mumbai:** PWD Shed. Gala no. 25/26, Ramchandra Bhatt Marg, Next to JJ Hospital Gate no. 2,
  Opp. Union Bank of India, Noorbaug, Mumbai-400009, Maharashtra, India
  Ph: 022-66661880/89   e-mail: mumbai@cbspd.com

Representatives

• **Hyderabad**	0-9885175004	• **Jharkhand**	0-9811541605	• **Nagpur**	0-9421945513
• **Patna**	0-9334159340	• **Pune**	0-9923910676	• **Uttarakhand**	0-9716462459

Printed at Chaman Enterprises, Delhi, India

Preface

This logbook has been designed keeping in mind the requirements of the new Competency Based Medical Education (CBME) curriculum.

Individual departments have the flexibility to decide the list of competencies to be included in this logbook and specify the maximum number of attempts allowed for each activity. Adequate space is provided to enter the details of the competencies and activities, the details of remedial training (if any), the rating for each attempt at the activity and the final decision of the faculty. The assessment scale has only two ratings, 'Scope for further improvement' and 'Satisfactory'; thereby emphasising on positive motivation for all students.

Sections on important topics from the subject have been designed as reflective portfolios with ample space for reflection writing by the student learners. Separate sections have also been designed for SBT (Simulation Based Teaching), AETCOM (Attitude, Ethics and Communication) and Integration.

Introduction

The Competency Based Medical Education (CBME) curriculum for undergraduate medical education was introduced in the academic year 2019–2020. The new curriculum has brought about a fundamental change in the system of medical education in our country. There is greater emphasis on alignment and integration of the various subjects, on the acquisition of specific competencies and essential skills and on the assessment 'for' learning. Maintaining a record of the activities conducted and the competencies and skills acquired is now a mandatory requirement.

This logbook aims to provide a ready format to record the activities, competencies and skills in **Pharmacology**. Combined with reflection writing, the records can be used for formative and continuous assessment of the learners as they progress through the year and onwards to Third Professional MBBS. We hope that this logbook will serve as a stimulus to encourage self-directed learning among undergraduate students.

Salient Features

1. Simple tabular format of the templates for recording the activities conducted and competencies and skills acquired
2. An assessment scale with only two ratings, Scope for further improvement and Satisfactory; thereby emphasising on positive motivation for all students
3. Flexibility to record the competencies decided by individual departments
4. Ample space in each row to record and assess all activities under a given competency
5. Reflective portfolios for important topics with encouragement of reflection writing and recording the details of assignments and assessments
6. Separate sections for SBT (Simulation Based Teaching), AETCOM (Attitude, Ethics and Communication) and Integration

Niket Verma
Poonam Agrawal
Deepti Chopra

Certificate 1

It is hereby certified that Ms./Mr. …………..…………….....……………………....., Roll No./University Registration No. ……………………………..……..., who is a student of IInd Professional MBBS at……………..…………………………….…….. (name of Medical College), has satisfactorily achieved all competencies (including certifiable competencies) and completed all assignments from Pharmacology mentioned in this logbook.

  She/He is eligible to appear for the IInd Professional MBBS University examinations in Pharmacology which will be conducted by …………………………………....….. (name of the affiliating university), from ……………….. to……………….. .

Signature of Faculty-incharge

Signature of Head of the Department

Signature of Principal/Dean of the College

Certificate 2

It is hereby certified that Ms./Mr. …………..…………….....……………………....., Roll No./University Registration No. ……………………………..……..., who is a student of IInd Professional MBBS at……………………………………………. (name of Medical College), has NOT achieved all competencies (including certifiable competencies) and/or completed all assignments from Pharmacology mentioned in this logbook.

  She/He is NOT eligible to appear for the IInd Professional MBBS University examinations in Pharmacology which will be conducted by ……………………....….. (name of the affiliating university), from ………………. to………………. .

Signature of Faculty-incharge

Signature of Head of the Department

Signature of Principal/Dean of the College

Contents

Section 1: Introduction to Pharmacology

Sr. No.	Competency number and description of the activity	Maximum number of attempts allowed for the activity	No. of attempts taken by the learner (with date of each attempt)	Any remedial training needed? (Yes/No) If yes then state the reason(s)	Rating 1. Scope for further improvement 2. Satisfactory (All attempts at the activity must be rated separately)	Final decision of faculty C– Completed N–Not completed	Feedback conveyed by faculty (Yes/No) Signature of faculty (with date)	Feedback received by learner (Yes/No) Signature of learner (with date)
	Introduction to Pharmacology							
1.								
2.								
3.								
4.								
5.								

Section 1: Introduction to Pharmacology

(This page may be used to record the salient points of the discussion as well as any activities, assignments or assessments on the topic)

Sub-topic: Date:

1. Please describe briefly what was discussed OR details of activity/assignment/assessment:

2. What did you learn from the discussion OR the activity/assignment/assessment:

3. Do you feel that the knowledge you have acquired will help you become a better doctor? Please explain in your own words.

Feedback Received (Yes/No):

Section 1A: History and Evolution of Pharmacology

(This page may be used to record the salient points of the discussion as well as any activities, assignments or assessments on the topic)

Sub-topic: Date:

1. Please describe briefly what was discussed OR details of activity/assignment/assessment:

2. What did you learn from the discussion OR the activity/assignment/assessment:

3. Do you feel that the knowledge you have acquired will help you become a better doctor? Please explain in your own words.

Feedback Received (Yes/No):

Section 1B: The Role of Pharmacology in Disease Management

(This page may be used to record the salient points of the discussion as well as any activities, assignments or assessments on the topic)

Sub-topic: Date:

1. Please describe briefly what was discussed OR details of activity/assignment/assessment:

2. What did you learn from the discussion OR the activity/assignment/assessment:

3. Do you feel that the knowledge you have acquired will help you become a better doctor? Please explain in your own words.

Feedback Received (Yes/No):

Section 2: General Pharmacology

Sr. No.	Competency number and description of the activity	Maximum number of attempts allowed for the activity	No. of attempts taken by the learner (with date of each attempt)	Any remedial training needed? (Yes/No) If yes then state the reason(s)	Rating 1. Scope for further improvement 2. Satisfactory (All attempts at the activity must be rated separately)	Final decision of faculty C– Completed N–Not completed	Feedback conveyed by faculty (Yes/No) Signature of faculty (with date)	Feedback received by learner (Yes/No) Signature of learner (with date)
	General Pharmacology							
1.								
2.								
3.								
4.								
5.								

Section 2: General Pharmacology

Sr. No.	Competency number and description of the activity	Maximum number of attempts allowed for the activity	No. of attempts taken by the learner (with date of each attempt)	Any remedial training needed? (Yes/No) If yes then state the reason(s)	Rating 1. Scope for further improvement 2. Satisfactory (All attempts at the activity must be rated separately)	Final decision of faculty C– Completed N–Not completed	Feedback conveyed by faculty (Yes/No) Signature of faculty (with date)	Feedback received by learner (Yes/No) Signature of learner (with date)
				General Pharmacology				
6.								
7.								
8.								
9.								
10.								

Section 2: General Pharmacology

Sr. No.	Competency number and description of the activity	Maximum number of attempts allowed for the activity	No. of attempts taken by the learner (with date of each attempt)	Any remedial training needed? (Yes/No) If yes then state the reason(s)	Rating 1. Scope for further improvement 2. Satisfactory (All attempts at the activity must be rated separately)	Final decision of faculty C– Completed N–Not completed	Feedback conveyed by faculty (Yes/No) Signature of faculty (with date)	Feedback received by learner (Yes/No) Signature of learner (with date)
				General Pharmacology				
11.								
12.								
13.								
14.								
15.								

Section 2: General Pharmacology

(This page may be used to record the salient points of the discussion as well as any activities, assignments or assessments on the topic)

Sub-topic: Date:

1. Please describe briefly what was discussed OR details of activity/assignment/assessment:

2. What did you learn from the discussion OR the activity/assignment/assessment:

3. Do you feel that the knowledge you have acquired will help you become a better doctor? Please explain in your own words.

Feedback Received (Yes/No):

Section 3: Clinical Pharmacology

Sr No.	Competency number and description of the activity	Maximum number of attempts allowed for the activity	No. of attempts taken by the learner (with date of each attempt)	Any remedial training needed? (Yes/No) If yes then state the reason(s)	Rating 1. Scope for further improvement 2. Satisfactory (All attempts at the activity must be rated separately)	Final decision of faculty C– Completed N–Not completed	Feedback conveyed by faculty (Yes/No) Signature of faculty (with date)	Feedback received by learner (Yes/No) Signature of learner (with date)
				Clinical Pharmacology				
1.								
2.								
3.								
4.								
5.								

Section 3: Clinical Pharmacology

Sr. No.	Competency number and description of the activity	Maximum number of attempts allowed for the activity	No. of attempts taken by the learner (with date of each attempt)	Any remedial training needed? (Yes/No) If yes then state the reason(s)	Rating 1. Scope for further improvement 2. Satisfactory (All attempts at the activity must be rated separately)	Final decision of faculty C– Completed N–Not completed	Feedback conveyed by faculty (Yes/No) Signature of faculty (with date)	Feedback received by learner (Yes/No) Signature of learner (with date)
				Clinical Pharmacology				
6.								
7.								
8.								
9.								
10.								

Section 3: Clinical Pharmacology

Sr. No.	Competency number and description of the activity	Maximum number of attempts allowed for the activity	No. of attempts taken by the learner (with date of each attempt)	Any remedial training needed? (Yes/No) If yes then state the reason(s)	Rating 1. Scope for further improvement 2. Satisfactory (All attempts at the activity must be rated separately)	Final decision of faculty C– Completed N–Not completed	Feedback conveyed by faculty (Yes/No) Signature of faculty (with date)	Feedback received by learner (Yes/No) Signature of learner (with date)
				Clinical Pharmacology				
11.								
12.								
13.								
14.								
15.								

Section 3: Clinical Pharmacology

(This page may be used to record the salient points of the discussion as well as any activities, assignments or assessments on the topic)

Sub-topic: Date:

1. Please describe briefly what was discussed OR details of activity/assignment/assessment:

2. What did you learn from the discussion OR the activity/assignment/assessment:

3. Do you feel that the knowledge you have acquired will help you become a better doctor? Please explain in your own words.

Feedback Received (Yes/No):

Section 4: Experimental Pharmacology

Sr. No.	Competency number and description of the activity	Maximum number of attempts allowed for the activity	No. of attempts taken by the learner (with date of each attempt)	Any remedial training needed? (Yes/No) If yes then state the reason(s)	Rating 1. Scope for further improvement 2. Satisfactory (All attempts at the activity must be rated separately)	Final decision of faculty C– Completed N–Not completed	Feedback conveyed by faculty (Yes/No) Signature of faculty (with date)	Feedback received by learner (Yes/No) Signature of learner (with date)
			Experimental Pharmacology					
1.								
2.								
3.								
4.								
5.								

Section 4: Experimental Pharmacology

Sr. No.	Competency number and description of the activity	Maximum number of attempts allowed for the activity	No. of attempts taken by the learner (with date of each attempt)	Any remedial training needed? (Yes/No) If yes then state the reason(s)	Rating 1. Scope for further improvement 2. Satisfactory (All attempts at the activity must be rated separately)	Final decision of faculty C– Completed N–Not completed	Feedback conveyed by faculty (Yes/No) Signature of faculty (with date)	Feedback received by learner (Yes/No) Signature of learner (with date)
			Experimental Pharmacology					
6.								
7.								
8.								
9.								
10.								

Section 4: Experimental Pharmacology

(This page may be used to record the salient points of the discussion as well as any activities, assignments or assessments on the topic)

Sub-topic: Date:

1. Please describe briefly what was discussed OR details of activity/assignment/assessment:

2. What did you learn from the discussion OR the activity/assignment/assessment:

3. Do you feel that the knowledge you have acquired will help you become a better doctor? Please explain in your own words.

Feedback Received (Yes/No):

Section 5: Routes of Drug Administration

Section 5: Routes of Drug Administration

Section 5: Routes of Drug Administration

(This page may be used to record the salient points of the discussion as well as any activities, assignments or assessments on the topic)

Sub-topic: Date:

1. Please describe briefly what was discussed OR details of activity/assignment/assessment:

2. What did you learn from the discussion OR the activity/assignment/assessment:

3. Do you feel that the knowledge you have acquired will help you become a better doctor? Please explain in your own words.

Feedback Received (Yes/No):

Section 5: Routes of Drug Administration

(This page may be used to record the salient points of the discussion as well as any activities, assignments or assessments on the topic)

Sub-topic: Date:

1. Please describe briefly what was discussed OR details of activity/assignment/assessment:

2. What did you learn from the discussion OR the activity/assignment/assessment:

3. Do you feel that the knowledge you have acquired will **help** you become a better doctor? Please explain in your own words.

Feedback Received (Yes/No):

Section 6: Drug Formulations and Drug Delivery Systems

(This page may be used to record the salient points of the discussion as well as any activities, assignments or assessments on the topic)

Sub-topic: Date:

1. Please describe briefly what was discussed OR details of activity/assignment/assessment:

2. What did you learn from the discussion OR the activity/assignment/assessment:

3. Do you feel that the knowledge you have acquired will help you become a better doctor? Please explain in your own words.

Feedback Received (Yes/No):

Section 6: Drug Formulations and Drug Delivery Systems

(This page may be used to record the salient points of the discussion as well as any activities, assignments or assessments on the topic)

Sub-topic: Date:

1. Please describe briefly what was discussed OR details of activity/assignment/assessment:

2. What did you learn from the discussion OR the activity/assignment/assessment:

3. Do you feel that the knowledge you have acquired will help you become a better doctor? Please explain in your own words.

Feedback Received (Yes/No):

Section 7: Antibiotic Stewardship

(This page may be used to record the salient points of the discussion as well as any activities, assignments or assessments on the topic)

Sub-topic: Date:

1. Please describe briefly what was discussed OR details of activity/assignment/assessment:

2. What did you learn from the discussion OR the activity/assignment/assessment:

3. Do you feel that the knowledge you have acquired will help you become a better doctor? Please explain in your own words.

Feedback Received (Yes/No):

Section 8: Pharmacovigilance and Adverse Drug Reaction Reporting Systems

(This page may be used to record the salient points of the discussion as well as any activities, assignments or assessments on the topic)

Sub-topic: Date:

1. Please describe briefly what was discussed OR details of activity/assignment/assessment:

2. What did you learn from the discussion OR the activity/assignment/assessment:

3. Do you feel that the knowledge you have acquired will help you become a better doctor? Please explain in your own words.

Feedback Received (Yes/No):

Section 8: Pharmacovigilance and Adverse Drug Reaction Reporting Systems

(This page may be used to record the salient points of the discussion as well as any activities, assignments or assessments on the topic)

Sub-topic: Date:

1. Please describe briefly what was discussed OR details of activity/assignment/assessment:

2. What did you learn from the discussion OR the activity/assignment/assessment:

3. Do you feel that the knowledge you have acquired will help you become a better doctor? Please explain in your own words.

Feedback Received (Yes/No):

Section 9: Pharmacogenomics and Pharmacoeconomics

(This page may be used to record the salient points of the discussion as well as any activities, assignments or assessments on the topic)

Sub-topic: Date:

1. Please describe briefly what was discussed OR details of activity/assignment/assessment:

2. What did you learn from the discussion OR the activity/assignment/assessment:

3. Do you feel that the knowledge you have acquired will help you become a better doctor? Please explain in your own words.

Feedback Received (Yes/No):

Section 9: Pharmacogenomics and Pharmacoeconomics

(This page may be used to record the salient points of the discussion as well as any activities, assignments or assessments on the topic)

Sub-topic: Date:

1. Please describe briefly what was discussed OR details of activity/assignment/assessment:

2. What did you learn from the discussion OR the activity/assignment/assessment:

3. Do you feel that the knowledge you have acquired will help you become a better doctor? Please explain in your own words.

Feedback Received (Yes/No):

Section 10: Prescription Writing

Practice Exercise in Prescription Writing

Practice Exercise in Prescription Writing

Practice Exercise in Prescription Writing

Practice Exercise in Prescription Writing

Practice Exercise in Prescription Writing

Practice Exercise in Prescription Writing

Section 10: Prescription Writing

(This page may be used to record the salient points of the discussion as well as any activities, assignments or assessments on the topic)

Sub-topic: Date:

1. Please describe briefly what was discussed OR details of activity/assignment/assessment:

2. What did you learn from the discussion OR the activity/assignment/assessment:

3. Do you feel that the knowledge you have acquired will help you become a better doctor? Please explain in your own words.

Feedback Received (Yes/No):

Section 10: Prescription Writing

(This page may be used to record the salient points of the discussion as well as any activities, assignments or assessments on the topic)

Sub-topic: Date:

1. Please describe briefly what was discussed OR details of activity/assignment/assessment:

2. What did you learn from the discussion OR the activity/assignment/assessment:

3. Do you feel that the knowledge you have acquired will help you become a better doctor? Please explain in your own words.

Feedback Received (Yes/No):

Section 11: Drug Labelling

Practice Exercise in Drug Labelling

Practice Exercise in Drug Labelling

Section 11: Drug Labelling·

(This page may be used to record the salient points of the discussion as well as any activities, assignments or assessments on the topic)

Sub-topic: Date:

1. Please describe briefly what was discussed OR details of activity/assignment/assessment:

2. What did you learn from the discussion OR the activity/assignment/assessment:

3. Do you feel that the knowledge you have acquired will help you become a better doctor? Please explain in your own words.

Feedback Received (Yes/No):

Section 11: Drug Labelling

(This page may be used to record the salient points of the discussion as well as any activities, assignments or assessments on the topic)

Sub-topic: Date:

1. Please describe briefly what was discussed OR details of activity/assignment/assessment:

2. What did you learn from the discussion OR the activity/assignment/assessment:

3. Do you feel that the knowledge you have acquired will help you become a better doctor? Please explain in your own words.

Feedback Received (Yes/No):

Section 12: P-Drug Concept

(This page may be used to record the salient points of the discussion as well as any activities, assignments or assessments on the topic)

Sub-topic: Date:

1. Please describe briefly what was discussed OR details of activity/assignment/assessment:

2. What did you learn from the discussion OR the activity/assignment/assessment:

3. Do you feel that the knowledge you have acquired will help you become a better doctor? Please explain in your own words.

Feedback Received (Yes/No):

Section 12: P-Drug Concept

(This page may be used to record the salient points of the discussion as well as any activities, assignments or assessments on the topic)

Sub-topic: Date:

1. Please describe briefly what was discussed OR details of activity/assignment/assessment:

2. What did you learn from the discussion OR the activity/assignment/assessment

3. Do you feel that the knowledge you have acquired will help you become a better doctor? Please explain in your own words.

Feedback Received (Yes/No):

Section 13: Calculation of Drug Dosage

Practice Exercise in Calculation of Drug Dosage

Practice Exercise in Calculation of Drug Dosage

Section 13: Calculation of Drug Dosage

(This page may be used to record the salient points of the discussion as well as any activities, assignments or assessments on the topic)

Sub-topic: Date:

1. Please describe briefly what was discussed OR details of activity/assignment/assessment:

2. What did you learn from the discussion OR the activity/assignment/assessment:

3. Do you feel that the knowledge you have acquired will help you become a better doctor? Please explain in your own words.

Feedback Received (Yes/No):

Section 13: Calculation of Drug Dosage

(This page may be used to record the salient points of the discussion as well as any activities, assignments or assessments on the topic)

Sub-topic: Date:

1. Please describe briefly what was discussed OR details of activity/assignment/assessment:

2. What did you learn from the discussion OR the activity/assignment/assessment:

3. Do you feel that the knowledge you have acquired will help you become a better doctor? Please explain in your own words.

Feedback Received (Yes/No):

Section 14: Drug Abuse and Drug De-addiction

(This page may be used to record the salient points of the discussion as well as any activities, assignments or assessments on the topic)

Sub-topic: Date:

1. Please describe briefly what was discussed OR details of activity/assignment/assessment:

2. What did you learn from the discussion OR the activity/assignment/assessment:

3. Do you feel that the knowledge you have acquired will help you become a better doctor? Please explain in your own words.

Feedback Received (Yes/No):

Section 14: Drug Abuse and Drug De-addiction

(This page may be used to record the salient points of the discussion as well as any activities, assignments or assessments on the topic)

Sub-topic: Date:

1. Please describe briefly what was discussed OR details of activity/assignment/assessment:

2. What did you learn from the discussion OR the activity/assignment/assessment:

3. Do you feel that the knowledge you have acquired will help you become a better doctor? Please explain in your own words.

Feedback Received (Yes/No):

Section 15: Vaccines

(This page may be used to record the salient points of the discussion as well as any activities, assignments or assessments on the topic)

Sub-topic: Date:

1. Please describe briefly what was discussed OR details of activity/assignment/assessment:

2. What did you learn from the discussion OR the activity/assignment/assessment:

3. Do you feel that the knowledge you have acquired will help you become a better doctor? Please explain in your own words.

Feedback Received (Yes/No):

Section 15: Vaccines

(This page may be used to record the salient points of the discussion as well as any activities, assignments or assessments on the topic)

Sub-topic: Date:

1. Please describe briefly what was discussed OR details of activity/assignment/assessment:

2. What did you learn from the discussion OR the activity/assignment/assessment

3. Do you feel that the knowledge you have acquired will help you become a better doctor? Please explain in your own words.

Feedback Received (Yes/No):

Section 16: National Health Programmes

National Health Programmes in India

National Health Programmes in India

Section 16: National Health Programmes

(This page may be used to record the salient points of the discussion as well as any activities, assignments or assessments on the topic)

Sub-topic: Date:

1. Please describe briefly what was discussed OR details of activity/assignment/assessment:

2. What did you learn from the discussion OR the activity/assignment/assessment:

3. Do you feel that the knowledge you have acquired will help you become a better doctor? Please explain in your own words.

Feedback Received (Yes/No):

Section 16: National Health Programmes

(This page may be used to record the salient points of the discussion as well as any activities, assignments or assessments on the topic)

Sub-topic: Date:

1. Please describe briefly what was discussed OR details of activity/assignment/assessment:

2. What did you learn from the discussion OR the activity/assignment/assessment:

3. Do you feel that the knowledge you have acquired will help you become a better doctor? Please explain in your own words.

Feedback Received (Yes/No):

Section 17: OTC (Over-the-Counter) Drugs

OTC Drugs

(This page may be used to record the salient points of the discussion as well as any activities, assignments or assessments on the topic)

Sub-topic: Date:

1. Please describe briefly what was discussed OR details of activity/assignment/assessment:

2. What did you learn from the discussion OR the activity/assignment/assessment:

3. Do you feel that the knowledge you have acquired will help you become a better doctor? Please explain in your own words.

Feedback Received (Yes/No):

Section 17: OTC (Over-the-Counter) Drugs

OTC Drugs

(This page may be used to record the salient points of the discussion as well as any activities, assignments or assessments on the topic)

Sub-topic: Date:

1. Please describe briefly what was discussed OR details of activity/assignment/assessment:

2. What did you learn from the discussion OR the activity/assignment/assessment:

3. Do you feel that the knowledge you have acquired will help you become a better doctor? Please explain in your own words.

Feedback Received (Yes/No):

Section 18: Essential Medicines

List of Essential Medicines

List of Essential Medicines

List of Essential Medicines

Section 18: Essential Medicines

(This page may be used to record the salient points of the discussion as well as any activities, assignments or assessments on the topic)

Sub-topic: Date:

1. Please describe briefly what was discussed OR details of activity/assignment/assessment:

2. What did you learn from the discussion OR the activity/assignment/assessment:

3. Do you feel that the knowledge you have acquired will help you become a better doctor? Please explain in your own words.

Feedback Received (Yes/No):

Section 18: Essential Medicines

(This page may be used to record the salient points of the discussion as well as any activities, assignments or assessments on the topic)

Sub-topic: Date:

1. Please describe briefly what was discussed OR details of activity/assignment/assessment:

2. What did you learn from the discussion OR the activity/assignment/assessment:

3. Do you feel that the knowledge you have acquired will help you become a better doctor? Please explain in your own words.

Feedback Received (Yes/No):

Section 19: Fixed Dose Combinations

(This page may be used to record the salient points of the discussion as well as any activities, assignments or assessments on the topic)

Sub-topic: Date:

1. Please describe briefly what was discussed OR details of activity/assignment/assessment:

2. What did you learn from the discussion OR the activity/assignment/assessment:

3. Do you feel that the knowledge you have acquired will help you become a better doctor? Please explain in your own words.

Feedback Received (Yes/No):

Section 19: Fixed Dose Combinations

(This page may be used to record the salient points of the discussion as well as any activities, assignments or assessments on the topic)

Sub-topic: Date:

1. Please describe briefly what was discussed OR details of activity/assignment/assessment:

2. What did you learn from the discussion OR the activity/assignment/assessment:

3. Do you feel that the knowledge you have acquired will help you become a better doctor? Please explain in your own words.

Feedback Received (Yes/No):

Section 20: Herbal Medicines

(This page may be used to record the salient points of the discussion as well as any activities, assignments or assessments on the topic)

Sub-topic: Date:

1. Please describe briefly what was discussed OR details of activity/assignment/assessment:

2. What did you learn from the discussion OR the activity/assignment/assessment

3. Do you feel that the knowledge you have acquired will help you become a better doctor? Please explain in your own words.

Feedback Received (Yes/No):

Section 21: Drug Regulations in India

(This page may be used to record the salient points of the discussion as well as any activities, assignments or assessments on the topic)

Sub-topic: Date:

1. Please describe briefly what was discussed OR details of activity/assignment/assessment:

2. What did you learn from the discussion OR the activity/assignment/assessment:

3. Do you feel that the knowledge you have acquired will help you become a better doctor? Please explain in your own words.

Feedback Received (Yes/No):

Section 21: Drug Regulations in India

(This page may be used to record the salient points of the discussion as well as any activities, assignments or assessments on the topic)

Sub-topic: Date:

1. Please describe briefly what was discussed OR details of activity/assignment/assessment:

2. What did you learn from the discussion OR the activity/assignment/assessment

3. Do you feel that the knowledge you have acquired will help you become a better doctor? Please explain in your own words.

Feedback Received (Yes/No):

Section 22: Drug Advertisement

(This page may be used to record the salient points of the discussion as well as any activities, assignments or assessments on the topic)

Sub-topic: Date:

1. Please describe briefly what was discussed OR details of activity/assignment/assessment:

2. What did you learn from the discussion OR the activity/assignment/assessment:

3. Do you feel that the knowledge you have acquired will help you become a better doctor? Please explain in your own words.

Feedback Received (Yes/No):

Section 23: Drug Development and Clinical Trials

Phases of Clinical Trials

Phases of Clinical Trials

Section 23: Drug Development and Clinical Trials

(This page may be used to record the salient points of the discussion as well as any activities, assignments or assessments on the topic)

Sub-topic: Date:

1. Please describe briefly what was discussed OR details of activity/assignment/assessment:

2. What did you learn from the discussion OR the activity/assignment/assessment:

3. Do you feel that the knowledge you have acquired will help you become a better doctor? Please explain in your own words.

Feedback Received (Yes/No):

Section 23: Drug Development and Clinical Trials

(This page may be used to record the salient points of the discussion as well as any activities, assignments or assessments on the topic)

Sub-topic: Date:

1. Please describe briefly what was discussed OR details of activity/assignment/assessment:

2. What did you learn from the discussion OR the activity/assignment/assessment:

3. Do you feel that the knowledge you have acquired will help you become a better doctor? Please explain in your own words.

Feedback Received (Yes/No):

Section 24: Miscellaneous Topics

(This page may be used to record the salient points of the discussion as well as any activities, assignments or assessments on the topic)

Sub-topic: Date:

1. Please describe briefly what was discussed OR details of activity/assignment/assessment:

2. What did you learn from the discussion OR the activity/assignment/assessment:

3. Do you feel that the knowledge you have acquired will help you become a better doctor? Please explain in your own words.

Feedback Received (Yes/No):

Section 24: Miscellaneous Topics

(This page may be used to record the salient points of the discussion as well as any activities, assignments or assessments on the topic)

Sub-topic: Date:

1. Please describe briefly what was discussed OR details of activity/assignment/assessment:

2. What did you learn from the discussion OR the activity/assignment/assessment:

3. Do you feel that the knowledge you have acquired will help you become a better doctor? Please explain in your own words.

Feedback Received (Yes/No):

Section 25: Recent Advances in Pharmacology

Section 25: Recent Advances in Pharmacology

(This page may be used to record the salient points of the discussion as well as any activities, assignments or assessments on the topic)

Sub-topic: Date:

1. Please describe briefly what was discussed OR details of activity/assignment/assessment:

2. What did you learn from the discussion OR the activity/assignment/assessment:

3. Do you feel that the knowledge you have acquired will help you become a better doctor? Please explain in your own words.

Feedback Received (Yes/No):

Section 26: Simulation Based Teaching (Skills Lab)

Simulation Based Teaching

(This page may be used to record the salient points of the discussion as well as any activities, assignments or assessments on the topic)

Sub-topic: Date:

1. Please describe briefly what was discussed OR details of activity/assignment/assessment:

2. What did you learn from the discussion OR the activity/assignment/assessment:

3. Do you feel that the knowledge you have acquired will help you become a better doctor? Please explain in your own words.

Feedback Received (Yes/No):

Section 26: Simulation Based Teaching (Skills Lab)

Simulation Based Teaching

(This page may be used to record the salient points of the discussion as well as any activities, assignments or assessments on the topic)

Sub-topic: Date:

1. Please describe briefly what was discussed OR details of activity/assignment/assessment:

2. What did you learn from the discussion OR the activity/assignment/assessment:

3. Do you feel that the knowledge you have acquired will help you become a better doctor? Please explain in your own words.

Feedback Received (Yes/No):

Section 26: Simulation Based Teaching (Skills Lab)

Simulation Based Teaching

(This page may be used to record the salient points of the discussion as well as any activities, assignments or assessments on the topic)

Sub-topic: Date:

1. Please describe briefly what was discussed OR details of activity/assignment/assessment:

2. What did you learn from the discussion OR the activity/assignment/assessment:

3. Do you feel that the knowledge you have acquired will help you become a better doctor? Please explain in your own words.

Feedback Received (Yes/No):

Section 26: Simulation Based Teaching (Skills Lab)

Simulation Based Teaching

(This page may be used to record the salient points of the discussion as well as any activities, assignments or assessments on the topic)

Sub-topic: Date:

1. Please describe briefly what was discussed OR details of activity/assignment/assessment:

2. What did you learn from the discussion OR the activity/assignment/assessment:

3. Do you feel that the knowledge you have acquired will help you become a better doctor? Please explain in your own words.

Feedback Received (Yes/No):

Section 27: Attitude, Ethics and Communication (AETCOM)

Sr. No.	Competency number and description of the activity	Maximum number of attempts allowed for the activity	No. of attempts taken by the learner (with date of each attempt)	Any remedial training needed? (Yes/No) If yes then state the reason(s)	Rating 1. Scope for further improvement 2. Satisfactory (All attempts at the activity must be rated separately)	Final decision of faculty C– Completed N–Not completed	Feedback conveyed by faculty (Yes/No) Signature of faculty (with date)	Feedback received by learner (Yes/No) Signature of learner (with date)
Attitude, Ethics and Communication (AETCOM)
1.								
2.								
3.								
4.								
5.								

Section 27: Attitude, Ethics and Communication (AETCOM)

Sr. No.	Competency number and description of the activity	Maximum number of attempts allowed for the activity	No. of attempts taken by the learner (with date of each attempt)	Any remedial training needed? (Yes/No) If yes then state the reason(s)	Rating 1. Scope for further improvement 2. Satisfactory (All attempts at the activity must be rated separately)	Final decision of faculty C– Completed N–Not completed	Feedback conveyed by faculty (Yes/No) Signature of faculty (with date)	Feedback received by learner (Yes/No) Signature of learner (with date)
	Attitude, Ethics and Communication (AETCOM)							
6.								
7.								
8.								
9.								
10.								

Section 27: Attitude, Ethics and Communication (AETCOM)

(This page may be used to record the salient points of the discussion as well as any activities, assignments or assessments on the topic)

Sub-topic: Date:

1. Please describe briefly what was discussed OR details of activity/assignment/assessment:

2. What did you learn from the discussion OR the activity/assignment/assessment:

3. Do you feel that the knowledge you have acquired will help you become a better doctor? Please explain in your own words.

Feedback Received (Yes/No):

Section 27: Attitude, Ethics and Communication (AETCOM)

(This page may be used to record the salient points of the discussion as well as any activities, assignments or assessments on the topic)

Sub-topic: Date:

1. Please describe briefly what was discussed OR details of activity/assignment/assessment:

2. What did you learn from the discussion OR the activity/assignment/assessment:

3. Do you feel that the knowledge you have acquired will help you become a better doctor? Please explain in your own words.

Feedback Received (Yes/No):

Section 28: Integration

Sr. No.	Competency number and description of the activity	Maximum number of attempts allowed for the activity	No. of attempts taken by the learner (with date of each attempt)	Any remedial training needed? (Yes/No) If yes then state the reason(s)	Rating 1. Scope for further improvement 2. Satisfactory (All attempts at the activity must be rated separately)	Final decision of faculty C– Completed N–Not completed	Feedback conveyed by faculty (Yes/No) Signature of faculty (with date)	Feedback received by learner (Yes/No) Signature of learner (with date)
					Integration			
1.								
2.								
3.								
4.								
5.								

Section 28: Integration

Sr. No.	Competency number and description of the Activity	Maximum number of attempts allowed for the activity	No. of attempts taken by the learner (with date of each attempt)	Any remedial training needed? (Yes/No) If yes then state the reason(s)	Rating 1. Scope for further improvement 2. Satisfactory (All attempts at the activity must be rated separately)	Final decision of faculty C– Completed N–Not completed	Feedback conveyed by faculty (Yes/No) Signature of faculty (with date)	Feedback received by learner (Yes/No) Signature of learner (with date)
					Integration			
6.								
7.								
8.								
9.								
10.								

Section 28: Integration

(This page may be used to record the salient points of the discussion as well as any activities, assignments or assessments on the topic)

Sub-topic: Date:

1. Please describe briefly what was discussed OR details of activity/assignment/assessment:

2. What did you learn from the discussion OR the activity/assignment/assessment:

3. Do you feel that the knowledge you have acquired will help you become a better doctor? Please explain in your own words.

Feedback Received (Yes/No):

Final Summary

Sr. No.	Section	Dates (dd/mm/yy)	Overall assessment (complete/incomplete	Signature of the faculty-incharge/HoD (with date)
Introduction to Pharmacology				
A	History and Evolution of Pharmacology			
B	The role of Pharmacology in disease management			
General Pharmacology				
Clinical Pharmacology				
Experimental Pharmacology				

Final Summary

Sr. No.	Section	Dates (dd/mm/yy)	Overall Assessment (complete/incomplete	Signature of the faculty-incharge/HoD (with date)
Routes of Drug Administration				
Drug Formulations and Drug Delivery Systems				
Antibiotic Stewardship				
Pharmacovigilance and Adverse Drug Reaction Reporting Systems				
Pharmacogenomics and Pharmacoeconomics				

Final Summary

Sr. No.	Section	Dates (dd/mm/yy)	Overall assessment (complete/incomplete	Signature of the faculty-incharge/HoD (with date)
	Prescription Writing			
	Drug Labelling			
	P-Drug Concept			
	Calculation of Drug Dosage			
	Drug Abuse and Drug De-addiction			

Final Summary

Sr. No.	Section	Dates (dd/mm/yy)	Overall assessment (complete/incomplete	Signature of the faculty-incharge/HoD (with date)
Vaccines				
National Health Programmes				
OTC (Over-the-Counter) Drugs				
Essential Medicines				
Fixed Dose Combinations				

Final Summary

Sr. No.	Section	Dates (dd/mm/yy)	Overall assessment (complete/incomplete	Signature of the faculty-incharge/HoD (with date)
Herbal Medicines				
Drug Regulations in India				
Drug Advertisement				
Drug Development and Clinical Trials				
Miscellaneous Topics				

Final Summary

Sr. No.	Section	Dates (dd/mm/yy)	Overall assessment (complete/incomplete	Signature of the faculty-incharge/HoD (with date)
Recent Advances in Pharmacology				
Simulation Based Teaching (Skills Lab)				
Attitude, Ethics and Communication (AETCOM)				
Integration				